The Pink Salt Weight Loss Trick

The 28-Day Ritual to Reclaim Energy, Melt Fat &
Balance Your Body Naturally

By [Dr. Jordan Vale]

Dr. Jordan Vale

This book is a work of nonfiction. The health information provided is based on the author's personal experience and research. It is not intended as medical advice. Readers should consult their healthcare provider before beginning any new health regimen.

For every woman who ever felt like her body was the enemy.

This book is your reminder: your body is wise, capable, and worthy of care.

Table Of Content

INTRODUCTION

Why This Book, Why Now

You don't need another crash diet. You don't need another supplement. And you definitely don't need to be told to "just try harder."

What you need — what we all need — is a way back to balance. Something simple. Gentle. Honest.

This book was written for the woman who feels like her body is no longer on her side. Who's tired of bloating, brain fog, and the kind of cravings that hit like a wave out of nowhere. Who's exhausted by the cycle of trying hard, then burning out. And who's finally ready to heal from the inside out — one morning at a time.

What You'll Learn Inside

In the next few pages, you'll discover:

The **science** behind Himalayan pink salt and why it's more than just hype

The exact **morning ritual** that supports digestion, hormones, and metabolism

How to reduce fatigue, curb cravings, and rebuild your rhythm — naturally

A full **28-day reset plan** that doesn't require dieting or perfection

Recipes, symptom trackers, and journal prompts to make this personal and sustainable

But this isn't just a book. It's a *reset button* — for your energy, your habits, and your relationship with your body.

Why It Works

Because it doesn't ask for everything.

It asks for *a few minutes each morning*. To hydrate. To breathe. To reconnect with your body. To start small — and let consistency do the heavy lifting.

You'll be surprised how powerful that can be.

So if you've been looking for a sign — to try again, to start over, to take your wellness back into your own hands — this is it.

Let's begin.

CHAPTER 1

: Welcome to Your Reset Journey

"This isn't just about weight. This is about balance, clarity, and energy — the kind that comes from deep within."

If you're reading this, chances are you've already tried a dozen things.

Maybe you've counted calories, fought cravings, downloaded the apps, watched the influencers. You've seen the number on the scale barely move. Or worse — it moved the wrong way. And deep down, you're wondering: "Why isn't this working anymore?"

You're not alone.

Thousands of women across the world are quietly asking that same question — especially in their 30s, 40s, and 50s. Hormones shift. Energy drops. Digestion slows. Stress spikes. And suddenly the wellness plans that *used to work...* don't.

That's where this journey begins. Not with guilt. Not with a strict diet. And definitely not with another false promise.

But with **a ritual**.

Why a Ritual — Not a Regimen?

Because rituals root us. They don't demand perfection. They meet us where we are — in our pajamas, in a rush, with a toddler on one arm or a meeting in five minutes.

This book gives you one small habit that can ripple outward into better digestion, less bloating, more energy, calmer cravings — and perhaps most important of all, a clearer connection to your own body.

Why Pink Salt?

Himalayan pink salt isn't magic — but it *is* mineral-rich, gentle on the body, and grounding in its simplicity. Combined with warm water, lemon, or nourishing herbs, it becomes more than a drink. It becomes a signal — to hydrate, to pause, to support your gut, your adrenals, and your rhythm.

You'll learn how to:

Use the Pink Salt Morning Ritual to reduce cortisol & support adrenal reset

Balance hydration and electrolytes naturally

Curb stress-based cravings

Track symptoms tied to thyroid and perimenopause

Rebuild consistency with your health — without burnout

What This Book Is (and Isn't)

This book **is**:

A 28-day natural reset designed for busy women

A hormone-supportive morning habit

A toolkit for cravings, energy, digestion, and emotional eating

A blend of modern science + ancient self-care

A safe space to start again

This book **isn't**:

A fad diet or starvation protocol

A miracle cure for hormone disorders

A weight loss gimmick with empty promises

How to Use This Book

Each day of the 28-day plan will include:

Your Morning Ritual (easy recipe)

A Science Note (1-minute insight)

A Micro-Journal Prompt (mental reset)

A Progress Tracker (energy, bloat, mood)

At the end of each week, you'll reflect, reset, and refine.

By Day 28, your habits will be rooted, your body more balanced, and your path forward — clearer than ever.

One Last Thing Before You Start

You don't need to be perfect.

Just begin.

This isn't about transformation in one giant leap. It's about reclaiming your energy one sip, one moment, one morning at a time.

You ready?

Let's begin.

CHAPTER 2

The Pink Salt Ritual & What It Actually Does to Your Body

"It's not magic—it's minerals, hydration, and a morning habit that resets everything else."

What Is the Pink Salt Ritual?

At its core, the Pink Salt Morning Ritual is simple:

1 glass of warm water + ½ tsp Himalayan pink salt
(Optional: lemon juice, a drop of apple cider vinegar, or a herbal add-in like ginger or mint)

You drink it **first thing in the morning**—before coffee, before food, before screens.

And yes… that's it.

But behind this simplicity lies a ripple effect that touches your digestion, hormones, cravings, hydration, and even your stress levels.

The Science Behind the Ritual

Let's bust a myth right away: No, pink salt won't melt belly fat on its own. But that doesn't mean it's useless. Quite the opposite.

Here's what **science actually says**:

1. Hydration at the Cellular Level

Overnight, your body becomes mildly dehydrated.

Pink salt contains trace minerals (magnesium, calcium, potassium) that help **water absorb better into your cells** than plain water alone.

This supports **adrenal health, electrolyte balance**, and **energy production**.

2. Digestive Kickstart

Warm salt water acts as a **mild stimulant for gastric juices,** supporting morning bowel movements and reducing bloating.

A hydrated digestive tract = smoother digestion = less gas and fatigue.

3. Craving Regulation

Cravings are often a sign of **mineral imbalance or cortisol spikes**.

Proper mineral intake (including salt) can help regulate adrenal hormones and reduce the intensity of emotional or stress-induced cravings.

4. Hormonal Support

Cortisol (your stress hormone) peaks in the morning.

Hydration and mineralization first thing helps **buffer that peak**, reducing stress load.

This is especially helpful for women dealing with **PMS, perimenopause, thyroid or adrenal imbalances**.

Safety First: The Truth About Sodium

Let's be responsible here.

Pink salt isn't a miracle—**and too much sodium is harmful.**

Safe Daily Dose: ½ tsp in the morning ritual = ~1000mg sodium (Still within range for most healthy adults when factored into your daily diet.)

Who should avoid or modify?

People with **high blood pressure, kidney conditions, or on low-sodium diets**

Pregnant women (consult doctor)

Anyone taking diuretics or thyroid meds (check for interactions)

We include alternate recipes in Chapter 6 for low-sodium and salt-free options.

Why Morning?

Your cortisol is naturally highest in the morning.

Your body is coming off an 8-hour fast.

Your digestion is most "primed" when rehydrated early.

Starting with a **simple, grounded action** sets the tone for the rest of your day.

This isn't just a recipe. It's a **reset ritual**.

Ritual → Routine → Reset

You're not just drinking salt water.

You're creating:

A new **identity** around healing

A new **pattern** your body can count on

A new **relationship** with health that starts with trust, not pressure

This tiny ritual carries big momentum.

CHAPTER 3

Understanding Cravings, Fatigue & Hormonal Chaos

"It's not just about willpower. It's about biology, burnout, and unmet needs."

Have you ever:

Eaten "clean" for days, only to binge on salty snacks or sweets by 8:00 p.m.?

Slept 7 hours and still woken up groggy and bloated?

Felt like no matter what you do, the weight won't budge — especially around your belly?

That's not laziness. It's not weakness. It's your **body trying to communicate**.

Let's decode the signals.

Why You Crave the Wrong Things at the Worst Times

Cravings aren't a lack of discipline — they're your body's **last-ditch attempt** to rebalance something it's missing.

Craving Sugar or Carbs?

Could be **unstable blood sugar, low magnesium**, or **emotional reward-seeking**

May also stem from **gut dysbiosis** or **adrenal fatigue**

Craving Salt or Crunchy Snacks?

May reflect **electrolyte depletion, low sodium**, or **stress-related cortisol spikes**

Your adrenals may be "screaming" for balance

Craving Chocolate or Dairy?

Often tied to **low magnesium, PMS**, or **serotonin deficiency**

Also may signal a need for **comfort and grounding**

Cravings aren't the problem. **Suppressing them without understanding them is.**

Why You're Always Tired (Even After Rest)

Fatigue is *not* just about sleep. It's about:

Mineral loss from stress (burning through magnesium, salt, potassium)

Poor digestion → Less nutrient absorption

Hormonal dysregulation (especially thyroid + adrenal imbalances)

Cortisol flattening — where your stress hormone is either *always high* or completely depleted

Pink Salt helps here in 3 subtle but powerful ways:

Replenishes sodium + trace minerals → supports **electrolyte and cellular energy**

Combats morning cortisol spikes → **reduces stress fatigue**

Supports hydration → better nutrient delivery and less brain fog

What Hormonal Imbalance Feels Like

Let's simplify the chaos.

Hormonal shifts can cause:

Unpredictable cravings

Weight gain around the belly

Irritability, anxiety, or sadness

Insomnia or early waking

Hair thinning, dry skin, or cold hands/feet

PMS, heavy periods, or irregular cycles

Most women experience at least *3 or more* of these — and they often go ignored.

This book helps you **track**, **identify**, and gently **rebalance**.

You're Not Broken — You're Overloaded

This ritual is a pattern interrupt. A way to press pause on the pressure. A small act of **consistency** that quiets the chaos.

Each day in your 28-day plan will help you:

Understand what your symptoms are really saying

Support your body without over-correcting

Feel more clear, grounded, and motivated — naturally

CHAPTER 4

The 28-Day Pink Salt Reset Plan (How It Works)

"Ritual meets rhythm. That's how real change sticks."

*You don't need another diet. You need a daily rhythm —
one that works with* your body, not against it.

That's why this isn't just a book. It's a **28-day
transformation ritual**—designed for real women, with real
lives, and real hormonal challenges.

No extremes. No starvation. No guilt. Just science-backed
simplicity that builds momentum.

The Core Goals of the Reset

Over the next 28 days, you'll:

Reduce bloating & digestive distress

Rebuild hydration & mineral balance

Curb cravings through daily ritual

Support hormone rhythm gently (thyroid, cortisol, estrogen)

Create consistency with 1 intentional action every morning

Your Morning Ritual Blueprint

Every day begins with:

1. The Pink Salt Morning Drink

8–10 oz warm filtered water

½ tsp Himalayan pink salt

(Optional add-ins: lemon, ACV, ginger, cayenne, or herbs)

Low-sodium? Use ¼ tsp or switch to **electrolyte tea** in Chapter 7.

2. Breath + Reflection

2–3 slow breaths

One grounding thought: *"I'm nourishing myself now."*

3. Micro Journal Prompt

Just one line: "This morning, my body feels…" (A daily self-scan builds body trust.)

4. Daily Symptom Tracker

Track: ☑ Bloating ☑ Energy ☑ Mood ☑ Cravings ☑ Sleep quality (from previous night)

Weekly Focus Breakdown

Week 1: Hydration & Digestion

Goal: Replenish minerals, reduce constipation/gas, ease stomach tension

Tools: Salt drink + gentle herbal teas + chew-your-food slow strategy

Week 2: Craving Reset

Goal: Address blood sugar & emotional hunger

Tools: Salt ritual + magnesium-rich food list + "pause & redirect" cravings chart

Week 3: Hormone Harmony

Goal: Support adrenal & thyroid recovery

Tools: Salt drink + journal prompts + cycle-awareness checklist

Week 4: Lifestyle Lock-In

Goal: Sustain results & build a "post-reset rhythm"

Tools: Salt habit + gratitude journaling + sleep prep + 3 bonus recipes

What You'll Need (Your Reset Toolkit)

Himalayan Pink Salt (fine-grain, food-grade)

1 Glass Mason Jar or Mug

Access to your 28-Day Printable Tracker (bonus link in final chapter)

Notebook or phone journal

Optional: lemon, ACV, herbal teas, calming playlist

Reminder: You Don't Need to Be Perfect

If you miss a day, you haven't failed. Just reset tomorrow. That *is* the ritual.

The real transformation happens when you:

Show up imperfectly

Stay curious

And keep going, even after a slip

This is a reset, not a test.

CHAPTER 5

Your Daily Reset Guide (28 Days of Ritual, Reflection & Rebalance)

"Consistency isn't built by doing more. It's built by doing less—repeatedly."

This is your day-by-day playbook.

Each day includes:

The Ritual — the drink recipe + mindful cue

Science Note — 1-sentence insight into what's happening in your body

Reflection Prompt — micro-journal or tracker cue

Optional Add-On — recipes, movement, or body-check suggestion

You can complete each day in **under 5 minutes.**

Let's begin.

WEEK 1: Reset Starts With Hydration & Digestion

DAY 1 ✓ **Ritual:** 8 oz warm water + ½ tsp pink salt Sip slowly, sitting down, phone off.

Science Note: This starts your digestive fire and begins rehydrating at the cellular level.

Reflection Prompt: "How does my belly feel *before* drinking this?"

Optional: Light stretching or 5-min walk post-drink.

DAY 2 ✓ Add 1 tbsp lemon juice to your ritual.

Lemon stimulates bile flow and aids liver detox pathways.

"What's one thing I want *less* of in my body today?"

Optional: Deep belly breathing, 3 slow inhales through the nose.

DAY 3 ✓ Try the ginger version: pink salt + lemon + pinch of powdered ginger.

Ginger reduces GI inflammation and bloating.

"Am I rushing through this, or letting it land?"

Optional: Chew each bite 20x today at one meal.

[...Day 4–7 will continue similarly, each with variations of salt, mindfulness, and light digestive tools.]

WEEK 2: Craving Control & Blood Sugar Reset

DAY 8 introduces cinnamon. DAY 9 adds optional pre-meal rituals. DAY 10 offers a craving tracker sheet. DAY 11 focuses on magnesium foods. DAY 12–14 builds self-trust and repeat power rituals.

WEEK 3: Hormone Support & Mood Regulation

DAY 15 brings back lemon & ginger + Epsom salt bath. DAY 16–17 introduces adrenal reset foods. DAY 18 encourages post-meal walking. DAY 19–21 focuses on emotional awareness, grounding practices, and gut-mood journaling.

WEEK 4: Lifestyle Integration & Long-Term Balance

DAY 22: Identify your "non-negotiables" for life after the 28-day plan. DAY 23–25: Emphasize rhythm: wake time, bedtime, mealtimes. DAY 26–27: Add 5-minute breathwork or gratitude journaling. DAY 28: Final reflection, habit lock-in, next steps planning.

CHAPTER 6

The Recipes — Detox Waters, Hormone Smoothies & Salt Variations

"Your ritual can taste good, feel good, and do good — all at once."

These recipes were designed to:

Support hydration, digestion, and cravings

Infuse beauty and joy into your wellness habits

Offer gentle hormone-balancing benefits using simple ingredients

Fit easily into busy schedules

You don't need a kitchen degree — just a glass, a spoon, and 3–4 minutes.

1. The Original Pink Salt Morning Drink

Ingredients:

8–10 oz warm (not hot) filtered water

½ tsp fine-grain Himalayan pink salt

Optional Add-ins:

1 tbsp fresh lemon juice (alkalizing + liver support)

¼ tsp raw apple cider vinegar (digestion + blood sugar)

Pinch of ginger powder (gut + inflammation)

1 drop food-grade peppermint oil or mint leaves (cooling + digestion)

When: First thing in the morning, before food or coffee.

2. The Brazilian Purple Elixir (Hormone-Balancing Smoothie)

Inspired by the viral trend, but upgraded for adrenal and thyroid health.

Ingredients:

½ cup blueberries (anti-inflammatory + estrogen balance)

½ banana (magnesium + cortisol support)

1 tbsp chia seeds (fiber + hormone detox)

½ tsp pink salt (electrolytes)

1 cup unsweetened coconut water (hydration + potassium)

1 scoop collagen peptides or plant protein (optional)

Blend until smooth. Drink within 30 mins of morning ritual.

3. Anti-Bloat Citrus Infusion

Ingredients:

10 oz cold water

Slices of lemon + cucumber + fresh mint

¼ tsp pink salt

Ice (optional)

Let infuse 5–10 mins before drinking. Sip throughout the morning.

4. Gut-Soothing Morning Mocktail

Ingredients:

8 oz water + 1 tsp pink salt

2 tbsp aloe vera juice (digestion + gut lining)

Splash of cranberry juice (liver + hormone detox)

Squeeze of lime

Stir well. Optional: add magnesium powder for PMS or constipation support.

5. Salt-Free Reset Option (For Low-Sodium Protocols)

Ingredients:

8 oz warm water

1 tbsp lemon juice

¼ tsp magnesium citrate powder

1 drop liquid trace minerals (like Concentrace)

Still delivers hydration + electrolyte benefit — without the sodium.

6. Hormone-Sync Smoothie for Cycle Support

Ingredients:
½ cup raspberries or blackberries

1 tbsp ground flaxseed (estrogen modulation)

½ tsp pink salt

1 tbsp almond butter (blood sugar + healthy fats)

1 cup unsweetened almond milk

Cinnamon to taste

Perfect in luteal or perimenopausal phases.

CHAPTER 7

Personalizing Your Reset for Hormones, Cravings & Special Needs

"One size fits no one. Real healing happens when you adjust, not restrict."

Your body isn't static. Hormones shift. Stress changes. Sleep fluctuates. That's why this reset isn't rigid — it's responsive.

This chapter shows you how to adapt your ritual to your phase of life, cycle, or needs. Whether you're dealing with PMS, perimenopause, cravings, low sodium requirements, or gut flare-ups — this plan flexes with you.

1. If You're Craving Everything All the Time
This likely means:

Stress eating (cortisol)

Blood sugar imbalance

Low magnesium or sodium

Emotional overwhelm

Reset Adjustments:

Add 1 tsp chia or psyllium to your morning ritual (slows cravings)

Include ¼ tsp cinnamon in salt drink (balances insulin)

Prioritize sleep → cravings drop 20–30% with 1 more hour

2. If You're in Perimenopause or Menopause

Your hormones are fluctuating daily. That means:

Lower estrogen → harder to detox

Lower progesterone → more bloating, anxiety

Slower metabolism + poor sleep

Reset Adjustments:

Use **lemon + pink salt + collagen** in morning ritual

Add magnesium citrate 1–2 hrs before bed

Introduce breathwork (Box Breathing 4-4-4-4) post-salt drink

3. If You're in Your Menstrual Cycle (Menstruating Women)

Cycle Phases Guide:

Menstrual (Days 1–5): Fatigue + need for iron/minerals → Stick to basic ritual with warm water + pink salt only

Follicular (Days 6–14): Energy rises → Add lemon + apple cider vinegar for metabolism boost

Ovulatory (Days 15–17): Inflammation risk → Use anti-bloat version (ginger + cucumber infusion)

Luteal (Days 18–28): Cravings increase → Add magnesium + cinnamon + adaptogenic tea

4. If You Have High Blood Pressure or Salt Sensitivity

Pink salt isn't inherently harmful, but you should reduce sodium if medically necessary.

Reset Modifications:

Use **¼ tsp or less** pink salt

Swap in **electrolyte herbal tea** (e.g. dandelion + lemon balm)

Use **coconut water + lemon + magnesium** instead of salt

5. If You Have Gut Issues (IBS, Bloating, Food Intolerances)

Salt can help, but additives might irritate the gut. Focus on **minimal ingredients**.

Reset Suggestions:

No lemon or vinegar for now

Use pink salt + water only for 3–5 days

Add aloe juice or chamomile if inflamed

Take ritual 30 min before any probiotic or gut supplement

6. Tracking Patterns: What to Watch For

Use your **Daily Tracker** to note:

Time of day when fatigue spikes

Cravings before or after certain meals

Digestive responses to specific ingredients

PMS symptom severity

Sleep quality after magnesium or salt variation

This is how *you build a custom health rhythm* that no diet could ever give you.

CHAPTER 8

The Psychology of Ritual — How Small Habits Create Big Change

"You don't need more willpower. You need better anchors."

Weight loss books often focus on food, calories, or workouts. But what drives real transformation — especially for women in their 30s, 40s, and 50s — is something deeper:

Emotional consistency

Nervous system calm

Identity-level change

That's the power of **ritual**.

What Is a Ritual (vs. a Routine)?

A routine is mechanical: wake, brush teeth, get dressed

A ritual is meaningful: sip, breathe, reflect, ground

Rituals combine *action* + *emotion* + *intention*. That's why your pink salt morning isn't just a drink — it's a cue, a commitment, a message to your body:

"I'm paying attention to you now."

The Habit Loop: How Ritual Becomes Automatic

Behavioral science shows that habits stick when they follow a **Cue** → **Action** → **Reward** loop.

Cue: Waking up

Action: Salt ritual (5-minute reset)

Reward: Mental clarity, digestive ease, self-pride

The more consistent this loop, the more effortlessly your brain begins to *expect* the ritual — and crave the reward.

Why Willpower Fails (And Rituals Don't)

Willpower is a finite resource. Rituals are renewable systems.

You don't need more motivation — you need fewer decisions. The salt ritual removes overwhelm by asking just one small thing at the start of the day. This creates *keystone momentum*, which spills into food choices, energy, and self-talk.

Ritual as Self-Respect

Many women have been told their body is a problem to be fixed. Ritual says: your body is worthy of care now — not "after you lose weight."

The pink salt reset becomes:

A **pause before panic**

A **replacement for negative self-talk**

A **daily dose of emotional safety**

It's not just a drink. It's identity work.

Your Morning Ritual + Anchor Prompt

Use this sentence each day *after* your salt ritual:

"Today, I nourish myself by _____."

Examples:

"...eating slowly and listening to my fullness."

"...asking for what I need."

"...saying no to what drains me."

Over time, this *rewires your identity* — from a woman who tries diets… to a woman who trusts herself.

CHAPTER 9

Real Women, Real Results — Stories from the Reset

"The ritual changed more than my body. It changed how I show up for myself."

Thousands of women have quietly transformed their health using this pink salt ritual.

Not because it's flashy. Not because it promises six-pack abs. But because it's simple, grounding, and real.

Here are just a few stories from women who've completed the 28-Day Reset — in their own words.

Madison, 39 – Perimenopause & Cravings

"I didn't expect much. But by Day 10, I noticed something wild: I stopped craving my nightly snack. I wasn't even fighting it — the urge just… wasn't there. My bloating dropped too, especially before my period. And mentally? I just felt calmer."

Her key changes:

Used pink salt + lemon daily

Added magnesium on Day 15

Paired ritual with morning journaling

Keisha, 44 – Postpartum Rebuild

"After baby #2, I felt disconnected from my body. The salt ritual gave me a reason to slow down and listen. It helped with water retention and mood. My energy came back first — the weight followed later."

Her key changes:

Did ritual while breastfeeding (with doctor's okay)

Used low-sodium version with ginger

Tracked energy and hydration — not weight

Renee, 52 – Hormonal Fatigue

"I didn't want another diet. I wanted peace. This gave me structure without punishment. By the end of Week 2, I was sleeping better, snacking less, and actually waking up with motivation."

Her key changes:

Added cinnamon in Week 2

Took Epsom salt baths in Week 3

Used 'pause and sip' ritual during stress peaks

Nita, 33 – Stress Eating & Gut Issues

"I used to binge after work. The pink salt ritual helped me *start* my day feeling in control, which stopped the spiral later. My digestion improved and my mood swings settled. I even started meal prepping again — and I hadn't done that in 2 years."

Her key changes:

Salt ritual + ACV version

Daily 5-minute morning journal

Switched to gut-soothing elixir on days 10–15

What You'll Notice (If You Stay Consistent)

Most women report:

Less bloating within 3–5 days

Reduced cravings by Day 7–10

Better energy and clearer skin by Week 3

A stronger sense of control and self-respect by Day 28

CHAPTER 10

After the Reset — How to Keep the Ritual Going for Life

"This isn't the end. It's your new beginning — just simpler, calmer, and more sustainable."

You've completed 28 days of consistency. 28 days of waking up, showing up, and tuning in.

Now what?

This chapter helps you turn the reset into a lifestyle — without pressure. Because sustainability is not about adding more — it's about *locking in what already works*.

The "Core Four" — What to Keep Going
Morning Salt Ritual

Keep it daily, or 4–5x/week if more realistic.

Mix in your favorite variation (lemon, ACV, ginger, etc.)

Micro Journaling

1 sentence each morning: "How do I feel?" or "What do I need today?"

Builds mindfulness and food-body awareness over time.

Weekly Reflection

Once a week, ask: *"What felt good this week? What didn't?"*

Use this to adjust food, stress, or sleep patterns.

Hydration Focus

Keep aiming for 60–80 oz of mineral-rich fluids per day.

Use detox waters, elixirs, teas, or your Purple Smoothie.

Monthly Ritual Rhythm

You don't have to stay in "reset mode" forever. But monthly check-ins help anchor progress.

Here's a sample monthly schedule:

Week 1: Full ritual + clean meals (great for PMS, cycle reset)

Week 2: Flexible mornings, but 3 salt drinks

Week 3: Add adrenal support (Epsom bath, magnesium, early bedtime)

Week 4: Low-stress rituals only (gentle walks, journaling, low-sodium elixirs)

If You Fall Off — Here's the 3-Day Mini Reset

Slipped out of rhythm? It's okay. Here's your soft reboot:

Day 1: Pink salt + lemon water + 1 quiet meal **Day 2:** Add Purple Smoothie + journaling + 10-minute walk **Day 3:** Morning salt + early bedtime + gratitude list

Then rejoin your normal routine.

What Real Sustainability Feels Like

It's not dramatic. It's not perfect. It's *gentle repetition*.

You'll trust your cravings less.

You'll trust your signals more.

You'll feel like wellness is *part of who you are*, not something you chase.

28 Days Tracker

Day 1

Date

Time of the Day

Ritual Done (Y/N)

Energy (1–5)

Bloating (1–5)

Cravings (1–5)

Notes:

_____

_____

_____

Day 2

Date

Time of the Day

Ritual Done (Y/N)

Energy (1–5)

Bloating (1–5)

Cravings (1–5)

Notes:

_____

_____

_____

Day 3

Date

Time of the Day

Ritual Done (Y/N)

Energy (1–5)

Bloating (1–5)

Cravings (1–5)

Notes:

_____

_____

_____

Day 4

Date

Time of the Day

Ritual Done (Y/N)

Energy (1–5)

Bloating (1–5)

Cravings (1–5)

Notes:

_____

_____

_____

Day 5

Date
Time of the Day
Ritual Done (Y/N)
Energy (1–5)
Bloating (1–5)
Cravings (1–5)
Notes:

_____

_____

_____

Day 6

Date
Time of the Day
Ritual Done (Y/N)
Energy (1–5)
Bloating (1–5)
Cravings (1–5)
Notes:

_____

_____

_____

Day 7

Date
Time of the Day
Ritual Done (Y/N)
Energy (1–5)
Bloating (1–5)
Cravings (1–5)
Notes:

_____

_____

_____

Day 8

Date
Time of the Day
Ritual Done (Y/N)
Energy (1–5)
Bloating (1–5)
Cravings (1–5)
Notes:

_____

_____

_____

Day 9

Date

Time of the Day

Ritual Done (Y/N)

Energy (1–5)

Bloating (1–5)

Cravings (1–5)

Notes:

_____

_____

_____

Day 10

Date

Time of the Day

Ritual Done (Y/N)

Energy (1–5)

Bloating (1–5)

Cravings (1–5)

Notes:

_____

_____

_____

Day 11

Date

Time of the Day

Ritual Done (Y/N)

Energy (1–5)

Bloating (1–5)

Cravings (1–5)

Notes:

_____

_____

_____

Day 12

Date

Time of the Day

Ritual Done (Y/N)

Energy (1–5)

Bloating (1–5)

Cravings (1–5)

Notes:

_____

_____

_____

Day 13

Date

Time of the Day

Ritual Done (Y/N)

Energy (1–5)

Bloating (1–5)

Cravings (1–5)

Notes:

_____

_____

_____

Day 14

Date

Time of the Day

Ritual Done (Y/N)

Energy (1–5)

Bloating (1–5)

Cravings (1–5)

Notes:

_____

_____

_____

Day 15

Date

Time of the Day

Ritual Done (Y/N)

Energy (1–5)

Bloating (1–5)

Cravings (1–5)

Notes:

_____

_____

_____

Day 16

Date

Time of the Day

Ritual Done (Y/N)

Energy (1–5)

Bloating (1–5)

Cravings (1–5)

Notes:

_____

_____

_____

Day 17

Date
Time of the Day
Ritual Done (Y/N)
Energy (1–5)
Bloating (1–5)
Cravings (1–5)
Notes:

_____

_____

_____

Day 18

Date
Time of the Day
Ritual Donc (Y/N)
Energy (1–5)
Bloating (1–5)
Cravings (1–5)
Notes:

_____

_____

_____

Day 19

Date

Time of the Day

Ritual Done (Y/N)

Energy (1–5)

Bloating (1–5)

Cravings (1–5)

Notes:

_____

_____

_____

Day 20

Date

Time of the Day

Ritual Done (Y/N)

Energy (1–5)

Bloating (1–5)

Cravings (1–5)

Notes:

_____

_____

_____

Day 21

Date
Time of the Day
Ritual Done (Y/N)
Energy (1–5)
Bloating (1–5)
Cravings (1–5)
Notes:

_____

_____

_____

Day 22

Date
Time of the Day
Ritual Done (Y/N)
Energy (1–5)
Bloating (1–5)
Cravings (1–5)
Notes:

_____

_____

_____

Day 23

Date

Time of the Day

Ritual Done (Y/N)

Energy (1–5)

Bloating (1–5)

Cravings (1–5)

Notes:

_____

_____

_____

Day 24

Date

Time of the Day

Ritual Done (Y/N)

Energy (1–5)

Bloating (1–5)

Cravings (1–5)

Notes:

_____

_____

_____

Day 25

Date

Time of the Day

Ritual Done (Y/N)

Energy (1–5)

Bloating (1–5)

Cravings (1–5)

Notes:

_____

_____

_____

Day 26

Date

Time of the Day

Ritual Done (Y/N)

Energy (1–5)

Bloating (1–5)

Cravings (1–5)

Notes:

_____

_____

_____

Day 27

Date
Time of the Day
Ritual Done (Y/N)
Energy (1–5)
Bloating (1–5)
Cravings (1–5)
Notes:

_____

_____

_____

Day 28

Date
Time of the Day
Ritual Done (Y/N)
Energy (1–5)
Bloating (1–5)
Cravings (1–5)
Notes:

_____

_____

_____

Printed in Dunstable, United Kingdom

67543417R00037